The Simple Secret of Successful Dieting and Weight-Loss That *Really Works!*

By B.T. Christopher

ISBN: 0-9817646-1-4
ISBN-13: 978-0-9817646-1-0

THE SIMPLE SECRET OF SUCCESSFUL DIETING AND
WEIGHT-LOSS THAT REALLY WORKS
Copyright 2012 by B.T. Christopher

St. Petersburg Press Inc. Po Box 21501
Sarasota, Florida 34276

WWW.SIMPLESECRETBOOK.COM

CONTENTS

INTRODUCTION

It seems that at any given time at least half of the adult population is trying to lose weight. Every year there are countless new diet/exercise books that come on the market. This is not one of them. Everyone already knows how to lose weight. The purpose of this book is to get you to actually do it.

Diet and exercise will cause you to lose weight. In order to change on the outside however, it is necessary to make a few small adjustments on the inside. It is my aim to help you to do that.

I have intentionally kept the book short and to the point (and even a bit corny in places). I have done-so to make it easy to read, understand, remember and put into practice. When you buy a book like this one, you are not buying words and paper, but the results you hope to gain from them. It is my belief that this book will supply the results that you seek

As you read, please try to keep an open mind. Some of the ideas here may seem a bit too simple to work. It has been my observation that simple ideas often work the best if you give them a try.

Also, to make things more simple, I have used the words "he" and "she" interchangeably. So if you are a "she", and it says "he" please don't take offense. The same goes for all of you "he" readers out there.

Good luck, and enjoy the book.

B. T. Christopher

Chapter 1
WHY MOST PEOPLE FAIL AT THEIR WEIGHT-LOSS PROGRAM

How many times in your life have you said "I am going to do "X""? It could be lose weight, exercise more, spend more time with the family, volunteer time to help those less fortunate, or whatever. Maybe you have made a New Year's resolution or two. "This year I will finally quit smoking once and for all." You want to do these things, you easily have the ability to do these things, you know that these things are good for you, and you know that you should do them.

But what happens? Time, and time again, these things somehow don't get done. These goals remain unattained. Year after year you remain stuck, virtually a prisoner of these seemingly inescapable habits and shortcomings.

Why in the world does this happen? Why does it seem so difficult to do the things we want to do and avoid doing the things we know we should not do and, more importantly, what can we do about it? How can we finally get our- selves to do what we want, and know that we should be doing?

Well, that's what this book is all about. Through many years of trial and error and diligent study, I have devised a simple but powerful method that works 100% of the time, <u>if you use it</u>.

Why you may have failed in the past

It is a well known fact that the vast majority of people who begin a weight-loss program will eventually re-gain whatever amount of weight, if any, they lose on the program. Many spend their lives going up and down in weight without ever achieving any permanent success. Maybe you even know someone like this.

There are, on the other hand, many folks who have actually succeed at losing weight, getting into shape, and staying that way for the rest of their lives. These successful people are in the minority, but they surely do exist. This is good news for the rest of us because they prove success is attainable! All we have to do is find out how they did it, and we can just copy them. When I say "find out how they did it" I do not mean what diet or exercise plan they followed. I mean find out *how they got themselves to follow it.*

Why are some people able to achieve their goals when many are not? What is the difference between the person who succeeds, and the one who doesn't? The answer, quite surprisingly, is not very much at all! We all possess the same basic equipment. We all have the same kind of brain, nervous system, heart, lungs, flesh, bones and muscles. We all have the ability to do it if we have to.

The basic difference is that the person who succeeds **wants to succeed**. And because they want to, they simply **choose** to. That is the simple and true fact. It always comes down to a choice. The successful minority chooses one way, and the unsuccessful majority chooses a different way.

Now, I know what you are thinking... "I want to lose weight! I don't like being overweight, I have been trying to slim down for years. I really do want to get into shape, and you can't tell me otherwise!"

I don't doubt it for a minute. I know you want to lose weight and maybe you have tried and even succeeded temporarily in the past. But at some point you made a choice to cheat on your diet "just this once" or skip a workout here and there and, before you knew it, you quit dieting and exercising altogether. Sound familiar to anyone?

I am, by no means, suggesting that you don't want it. What I am saying is that there have been times when you wanted to eat the foods and do the things that lead to weight gain more than you wanted your goal. Everybody wants to be lean and healthy, not everybody wants to do the things that will get them there.

Think of the state of "wanting something" as one of those old-fashioned scales. You probably have seen one at one time or another. They have two trays on opposite sides suspended from a beam with a hinge in the middle like a seesaw.

There is an arrow that points towards the side that has the most weight on it. They are called apothecary scales because they used to be used in pharmacies in the old days. If he wanted to measure half an ounce of some medicine, for example, a pharmacist would place a one-half ounce weight on one side of the scale and begin to add the medicine to the other side until the arrow was in the middle indicating the amount was equal to the weight on the other side. This type of scale is similar to our decision-making process. If we take 49 and 1/2 pounds and put it on one side of the scale representing our desire to lose weight, and 50 pounds on the other side representing our desire to overeat and avoid exercise, the needle would tip towards the side with the 50 pounds every time. Even though the side with our desire to lose weight has 49 and 1/2 pounds on it, it was just slightly outweighed by the other side. Even though the difference was slight, it was enough to make the scale tip to the heavier side and cause us decide to overeat. The difference was small, just like the difference between the successful dieter and the one who is unsuccessful.

The good news is that all we have to do is either take a little weight from the "desire to over-eat" side of our imaginary scale or add a little weight to the "desire to lose weight" side. But the best way is to do both at the same time. The goal of this book is to help you to tip the scale to the correct side.

You <u>can</u> succeed!

Some of you might be thinking that the successful dieter has more "willpower" than you do, or maybe that they were born with some special quality that you were not. This is not the case at all. They stayed with it because they chose to. They chose to because they wanted to. It does not take any willpower to do the things that you **want to do**. Nobody has to force themselves to do the things they enjoy doing.

This may be hard for some people to believe, but there are those who actually like to eat healthy, low-calorie foods. There are also some who dislike ice cream! The world does contain many folks who prefer exercise to lounging around the house.

For people like this, staying in shape is not a struggle. They don't have to force themselves to do the things that result in a lean and healthy body, they **want** to do them. Their imaginary decision making scale is always tipped in the direction of eating right and exercising.

Let's play a little game. Let's pretend you've been on your diet for a month or two and you have lost 20 pounds or so. Everything is going fine until your husband's (or wife's) birthday party. You were good and stayed on your diet all the way through the celebration until the cake came out. It was double chocolate (your favorite). You could almost taste it! Your mouth watered with anticipation and desire, but you remembered your diet and you didn't have any. After the party is over, and the people have gone home and everyone in the house has gone to sleep, you can't seem to get the thought of that cake out of your mind. You remember there is still a piece left over. You can't stand it anymore, so you sneak out of bed and make your way to the kitchen to get that piece. "I've been good all month, one piece can't hurt" you think. You are just about to dig in to the cake when, suddenly, a masked man appears in your kitchen with a big gun! He points his gun at you and says "If you eat that cake I will shoot you in both of your knee caps!"

Do you eat the cake? What a silly question right? Of course not! Are you crazy? You like chocolate cake but it's not worth getting shot over. What happened? One second ago you were going to eat the cake and now you're not.

You made choice! There was 10 pounds on the "eat" side of the imaginary decision-making scale, and there was 1000 pounds on the "don't eat" side. You could eat the cake and get shot, or you could not eat the cake and not get shot. You wisely chose not.

You might say "I had no choice." I say that you certainly did have a choice. What you really mean is that the choice was so obvious that it was easy to decide. You didn't even have to think about it!

I know that this situation is unlikely to come up in real life, and I don't suggest you hire a hit-man to follow you around all day and threaten to shoot you if you should go off your diet (although it would work!) What my little story does prove is that you have the ability to stay on your diet if you simply choose to! The person who succeeds uses the same power of choice (that I have just proven to you that you possess) to stay on their diet. They choose to!

The easy way

It is natural and normal for people to look for the easy way to do things. This has a bad sound to it, but it is mostly a good thing. It is this quality that is responsible for all the progress mankind has ever made! Most of mankind's greatest inventions were a result of his natural desire to find an easy way to do something. The caveman got tired of carrying heavy loads around, so he looked for the easy way and invented the wheel!

The trouble with this is when we mistake the easy way for the hard way, or even the impossible way and make incorrect choices based on this faulty perception.

You will always make the correct choices in life if you simply learn to recognize and avoid the mistakes in your thinking that make the easy way look like the hard way, and the hard way look easy. The path of least resistance usually turns out to be the path of most resistance.

Stop relying on what doesn't work

Imagine if someone handed you a treasure chest with a big padlock on it. And he handed you a key ring with 10 keys, and one of the keys was sure to open the lock. So you try the first key and it doesn't open the lock, what do you do? Simple, you keep trying different keys until you find the one that opens the lock, don't you? You wouldn't just keep trying the same one over and over, would you?

Sadly, this is the approach most people have toward weight loss. They go about it the same way that has failed them in the past, and then they are surprised and disappointed when they fail again.

This book is the key that will open the lock to successful weight loss once and for all.

One key that doesn't work

How many times in our lives have we heard it said that all we need to do to stay on our diet is to use "willpower" and "self-discipline"? We try, and try again, to develop these two magic traits in ourselves so that we may finally find success on our diets. Just like the lock and key example, we try over and over and they never work, so we assume that there must be something wrong with us.

There isn't anything wrong with you! You work just fine. You are not broken. The reason these two keys (willpower and self-discipline) don't work is because they represent pain in the here and now. Look at the word discipline. What feelings does it conjure up in you? For me it means **punishment** and **pain**.

When I was a kid in school and I got into trouble I would get "disciplined" by the teacher. This meant only one thing...pain, physical and emotional. Over the years I learned to try to avoid the pain of discipline at all costs. There is no way I'm going to do that "discipline" stuff to myself! I've grown kind of fond of myself over the years. So fond in fact, that I want myself to feel goodness, not discipline. Not only do I want to feel goodness, and not feel badly, I want to feel this way right now! Can you relate to this feeling?

Self-discipline does not work because it goes against our nature. People fail at weight-loss because they try to fight human nature. This book is definitely not about developing self-discipline. It is about succeeding by using the natural traits we already have within ourselves right now. We are going to learn to use human nature to our advantage, rather than try to fight with it.

Shift gears to go in the right direction

What is the difference between a car that is going forward and a car that is going in backwards? The answer is nothing. Both cars are the same. They both have four wheels, an engine that powers them, and a transmission that delivers power from the engine to the wheels. The engine always turns in the same direction whether the car is going forward or backwards. If your car is going backwards, and you wish for it to go forward, you don't try to change the direction in wich the engine is turning, do you? No, of course not, you simply shift gears, and the transmission converts the power of the engine (that's always turning in the same direction) to the wheels to make the car move forward.

I tell you this because the situation is so similar to that of the successful dieter and the unsuccessful dieter. They (the 2 dieters) are both the same. They both have the same basic equipment. They have the same body, the same brain, digestive system, heart, lungs, bones, muscles, emotions and feelings. Like the two cars, one uses its power to move forward and other one uses its power to move backwards. And just like the two cars, all that the unsuccessful dieter has to do to start moving in the direction they want is to simply shift gears and use the power that is already there.

It would be silly to go against our nature to be successful with our program, just as it would be to try to get our car's engine to run backwards to make the car go forward. Yet this is exactly the same approach that the unsuccessful dieters try to use over and over to no avail. They set goals for themselves and try to reach them by using willpower and self-discipline. It seems like it should work, and sometimes it does, temporarily. But using willpower and self-discipline is like treading water, eventually we can't do it anymore, and we become tired and weak and we sink.

You can do this. You are not broken. You have all equipment you need for success. Up until now you have been misdirecting your power. I will show you how to use your power correctly. This is the key that will finally open the lock your treasure chest.

Key Points:

-There is no difference between the person who succeeds and you. The only difference is in the choices that you make.

-The successful dieter chooses to eat right and exercise because she wants to, (<u>more</u> than she wants not to) at that point in time.

-You have the same power to choose.

-People want the easy way. They want to avoid pain and feel good now.

-Willpower and self-discipline will fail eventually because they go against human nature.

Chapter 2
WEAK VERSUS STRONG

Every one of us has within himself a weak side and a Strong side. The weak side wants us to do what it thinks feels good now. Some of these activities might include; oversleeping, goofing-off, watching too much television, overeating, smoking, drinking to excess, using drugs, indulging in debauchery, gambling, squandering money, acting selfishly, betraying people etc. But what it wants is always bad for us in the long run.

The Strong side, on the other hand, wants us to do what we know is right, even though we might not feel like doing it now. We say that we will do it "someday" but that day never comes. We know we should do these things, we know what is right and good for us, but rarely do we follow-through. Some examples would include things like; exercising, eating properly, going the extra mile at work or in our personal relationships, saving and investing our money, working on personal development, reading and learning more, developing our minds and spirits. All of the things that will, without any doubt, benefit our lives and the lives of those around us. We know we should not do things like smoke, drink, overeat, use drugs, gamble etc. because they will, most certainly, harm us and destroy our lives and the lives of those around us. We tell ourselves "we can quit any time we want to" (and we can if we choose to) but that "any time" never comes.

In between these two opposing sides of our makeup there presides a "judge." Her job is to decide which side, weak or Strong, we are going to let have control of our actions now, NOW being the key word (more on this later).

Because we have two opposing sides and a judge, our decision-making process can be likened to a court of law. I will use this comparison throughout the book to illustrate the way in wich we make our choices as we go about our daily activities.

How many times in your life has your judge decided in favor of the weak side? In my own life it has gone that way many more times than I care to remember. It all started when I was a small boy. When it came time to do my homework, there was usually something good on TV. My little judge would be persuaded by my weak side and decide that we can do our homework later, there will be plenty of time for homework in the future, but there is something good on TV **now**. But most of the time "later" never came. I would go to school without my homework, I would get into trouble at school, my parents would find out about it, and I would get into even more trouble at home.

Did I ever learn my lesson? Yes, many times! Did my little judge ever change the way he made his decisions? No, not at all! It just seemed to make him even more likely to choose to give-in to the weak side the next time around.

Maybe some of you have experienced a similar situation regarding food? "I'll start my diet after the holidays but I'm going to eat this pumpkin pie, ice cream and cake now." Or "I will go to the gym next week, but I have to watch THE JUDGE JUDY SHOW now." Does this sound familiar to anybody?

Why does the weak side always seem to get his way? How is it that the judge always seems to decide in his favor, even though she knows that it will harm us in the long run? What kind of incompetent judge are we dealing with here anyway?

The reason the weak side wins most of the time in our imaginary courtroom is because he has a better lawyer! The weak side is able to sway the judge to decide in his favor because he is able to convince her that she should do so, and that this is the right decision for now! (And he is certainly not above using trickery, deception, and even false evidence to do so!)

The Strong side, however, has a bad lawyer. His argument is always the same…"I am right. Everybody knows my way will benefit us the most in the long run. Even though it might seem to be a bit uncomfortable now, this is what we should do or not do."

This is not a very persuasive argument in the eyes of the judge. The Strong side relies only on logic to make his point. The weak side uses emotion, which is by far a more effective tool.

The weak side's argument is something like this… "Forget about down-the-road, this will make us all feel good now! It will even make the judge feel good now. My way is the *easy way*."

The judge tends to go along with this type of approach because, like most of us, she makes most decisions based on feelings and emotions. The weak side knows this, and uses it to his advantage again and again.

Every time the judge decides in favor of the weak side, it makes her that much more likely to decide in his favor the next time around. When the two sides get to court again the next time to decide what to do, the judge says "I have heard both arguments before and I stick by my original decision." She then bangs her gavel, says "case dismissed," and it's another victory for the weak side. Eventually the case doesn't even get to court, and the weak side wins automatically. His winning becomes a habit.

Think back to a time in your life when your judge let the weak side have his way. What happened? Did it ever help you in the long run? Imagine if you had done what your strong side had wanted you to do in that situation. Wouldn't that have led to a better outcome and ultimately made your life *easier* in the long run? The seemingly "easy way" is really the hard way, and the seemingly "hard way" is really the easy way. The weak side uses trickery to make this seem like the other way around (more on this in the next chapter.)

Still another dimension of the weak versus strong conflict is the fact that the more times we choose to be weak, the harder it becomes to choose to be Strong in the future. But the more times we choose to be Strong, the easier it becomes to choose to be Strong in the future until it becomes automatic, and we don't have to think about it. This is the state we are trying to achieve.

<u>Strong+Strong+Strong=Power
weak+weak+weak=powerless</u>

Think of it like this... if you were trying to make a strong rope out of thread, each time you add a piece of thread to your rope it gets a little bit stronger. If you take a piece of thread away, it gets weaker. Every time our judge rules in favor of our Strong side, we get stronger. Eventually being Strong will become automatic. Temptation will become a thing of the past. You will turn into one of those people who like to eat the right foods. Your desire for junk food will disappear. Your inner conflict will be no more. Exercise will become a priority. You will do the things that you know you should do because you like to do them.

All this will happen because your judge chose to rule in favor of the Strong side now.

Key Points:

-Everyone has a weak side and a Strong side.

-The weak side wants to do things that feel good now but will harm us in the future.

-The Strong side wants to do what will benefit us most in the future but might not seem to feel good now.

-There is a "judge" that makes the final decision of which side to give control of our actions.

-Every time we act in accordance with the weak side we get a bit weaker.

-Each time we act in accordance with the Strong side we get stronger.

Chapter 3
HOW THE WEAK SIDE USES LIES TO PERSUADE THE JUDGE

In the last chapter I compared the decision making process to a court of law. Keeping with that metaphor, in this chapter we will examine some of the ways the weak side manages to get the judge to do the things he wants.

The weak side is very clever and persuasive. He knows how to manipulate the judge, like a con artist does to separate his victims from their hard-earned money. Here are some of the tricks. Have you fallen for any of them in the past?

Self-image

Each one of us has a picture of himself in his mind. It's not only a picture, but a description of one's traits, characteristic's, talents and abilities, shortcomings, likes, dislikes etc. When we think of ourselves or describe ourselves to others we refer to this picture. This picture is known as our self-image, and it holds a lot of power over our lives. It is how we see ourselves. If we try to act in a way that is in conflict with our self image, we feel pain and uneasiness. The subconscious mind says "this is not normal," so it does everything it can to get us back to normal, as measured against our self-image.

This is a good system if we have a positive self-image, but it can be disastrous if our self-image is a negative one. Let's take the overweight person for example. In many cases they have been this way for years, maybe even their entire lives. So what happens? They develop the self-image of a "fat" person. They have nothing else to go by, as they have always been that way, so naturally they see themselves as a fat person. If they decide that they wish to lose weight, their self-image may stop them before they even get started. If they do begin to lose weight, instead of feeling good about themselves, they feel like something "isn't right" and before they know it the diet and exercise plan goes out the window and they are right back to "normal" as compared to their self-image.

The same thing happens in reverse to the thin person. They have always been thin. That is "normal" in their self-image. If they start to put on a few pounds, and their clothes start to get tight, that's "not normal" and they feel uncomfortable, both physically and mentally. So they do what is needed to get back to "normal," as compared to their self-image. As you can see, your self-image can either work for you or against you.

When the weak side is trying to persuade our judge to decide to let us cheat on our diet, or skip our workouts, or engage in any other weak behavior, he will use as evidence the self image.

In our imaginary court of decision making, the weak side's case might sound like this…"Your Honor, I call into evidence the self-image. As you can plainly see, the self-image is FAT! He always has been fat. If we were to get into shape, and lose weight, that would be wrong, it would violate the self-image. We must remain fat so that everything can stay "normal." I ask you Judge, in light of this evidence, that we eat this bag of potato chips and drink this 2 liter bottle of soda now so that we may remain normal!"

It sounds kind of funny, doesn't it? Maybe even a bit ridiculous. But this is pretty close to what goes on in our heads, even though we are not consciously aware of it. We have this mental picture of ourselves, which we firmly believe is 100% true and accurate. Something comes along to threaten our sense of what's "normal," or our unconscious sense of the way that things are supposed to be. This causes us to experience mental anguish or a general feeling of discomfort. We want to avoid this feeling, so we do something (in this case eat potato chips and drink soda) to ensure things stay the same.

Fear

Like the self-image, fear is a two-edged sword. It can either help us, or it can harm us. Fear is a survival mechanism. Surely without fear, mankind would not have survived for so many years, which is why it is so deeply ingrained in each of us. Even animals use fear to survive. Have you ever seen the face of a rabbit being chased by a dog? That is the face of fear. But if he wasn't afraid of the dog, the rabbit wouldn't run away, and the dog would kill him. His fear, unlike many of ours, is totally justified.

Fear and weakness go hand-in-hand. The more in a state of weakness you are, the more things you fear. And the more you fear, the weaker your state becomes. The weak side loves to use fear to sway the judge to decide in his favor, because fear is so powerful an emotion.

How many times in our lives have you or I not gotten, or failed to go after what we wanted because of fear? We did not get what we wanted because our weak side persuaded the judge to choose to "play it safe" with an argument like this… "Judge, if we go ahead and do this thing, there is no telling what kind of tragedy will befall us. We have never done this before. It will most likely cause us pain, even death, if we tried. We may lose all of our friends and be cursed with bad luck. We must act

38

prudently and avoid this thing. We must retreat back to where we were. It might not have been perfect, but we were used to it. At least we knew what to expect there. We had some level of comfort."

The weak side loves to live in the "comfort zone." The comfort zone may be thought of as a thermostat in your home. If the thermostat on your wall is set for 72° and it begins to get hotter outside, the air conditioner is automatically turned on until it brings the temperature back to 72°. If it gets too cold outside, the heat comes on and warms us back up to 72°... back to normal.

Each of us has their own built-in comfort zone that governs all areas of our life, not just our weight.

Let's look at the golfer, for example. For those of you not familiar with the sport, every golf course has a "par" rating. For most 18-hole golf courses, the par is 72. That number represents how many strokes (swings at the ball) a player is supposed to have to put the ball into the hole 18 times. If you can play 18 holes of golf, and only hit the ball 72 times, you will have played "par golf" or "parred the course." Some of the holes are longer (farther away from where you start) and you are allowed five strokes. There are some shorter holes where you allowed three. On most average holes they allow you four. To do this successfully is much more difficult than it sounds (take it from someone who has tried many times!). Only a very small minority of golfers, perhaps 1 or 2%, can play par golf. These players are known as "scratch golfers." The rest of us have what is called a "handicap." A handicap in golf is the number of strokes that must be deducted from one's average score to equal par. For example, if it normally takes me 82 strokes to play 18 holes, and par is 72, we would say that I was a 10 handicap (82-10=72). If I was playing against a scratch player, he would have to give me 10 strokes, a head-start if you will, to make us even. If I shoot 80 and he shoots 72, I would win because of my handicap (80-10=70).

This is a good system for golf because it allows players of all skill levels to play together on an even field. The problem, though, is that some players identify with their handicap. They come to believe it is "set in stone." Their handicap becomes part of their comfort-zone.

Let's imagine, for instance, on the first three or four holes, our 10 handicap golfer manages to make par. Instead of feeling happy that he is playing so well, his comfort zone says "this isn't normal." His friends notice he is playing better than usual and they start to make comments to him. "Hey Bob" they might say "have you been taking lessons?" This makes Bob feel uncomfortable and his comfort zone might think "They are right! You are a 10 handicapper. This is not how you play." And before you know it, Bob starts playing poorly to compensate for his good start. By the time he is done Bob scores his usual 82. In golf, as in life, a player's score will most times match his comfort zone.

I am sure that you have read about, or heard stories of people who were financially broke for many years and suddenly got a big pile of money. Maybe they won the lottery or got an unexpected inheritance. You would think these people would be set for life, but what happens most of the time is that they wind up poor again in a surprisingly short period of time. Why is this? You guessed it! They still have the comfort zone of a poor person. Being rich wasn't normal to them, so they found a way to lose all of their money quickly, and got themselves back to normal.

Just like the golfer and the lottery winner, the unsuccessful dieter is being held back by their comfort zone. When a person is overweight, on some level, they learn to get used to it. The body does not change as quickly as the mind, so they adapt. Like the self-image, they develop the comfort zone of the fat person. If they start to lose weight, they may begin to feel like something isn't right. This is uncharted territory. Others might begin to treat them differently. When they look in the mirror they see a stranger looking back at them. So just like the golfer and the lottery winner they unconsciously begin to sabotage themselves. They cheat on their diet. They stop exercising. And soon they are right back in their comfort zone. It's like the feeling you get when you come home from a vacation. "Hawaii was nice, but good old Greenland (with 6 feet of snow on the ground) is home! I was born here and I will die here. It's where I belong."

Pain

Everyone knows what physical pain is, and just like fear it is an important survival mechanism. A child who puts his hand on a hot stove for the first time feels pain and learns not to do that in the future. We all learn to avoid pain.

In addition to physical pain, we humans also experience emotional pain. If someone insults us and hurts our feelings we feel a certain amount of emotional pain. If a husband or wife leaves us for another, we feel pain. And just like that child with the hot stove, we learn to avoid this kind pain too.

The weak side can't take even the slightest bit of pain, physical or emotional. He is a wimp! "Judge" he wines, "I can't go to the gym today. Exercise equals pain!" Or "I'm hungry! I want pizza! The lack of pizza equals pain!" Weak wants to get himself as far away from what he thinks is pain as he possibly can. He wants pleasure, and he wants it now. To him diet equals pain. Exercise equals pain. The way he sees it, excess amounts of the wrong kind of food and inactivity equal pleasure. He feels so sure about this that he is able to persuade the judge to decide his way due to his enthusiasm. As I said before, weak has a good lawyer.

The future

This is one of the weak side's favorite tricks, and usually his last resort. This is when he knows he is wrong, and none of the usual arguments work. He agrees with the Strong side. We should do what we know is right, but we should do in the future. Not now, but someday.

This is the same tactic some parents use on their children to placate them, isn't it? Maybe yours used it on you when you were little. "Mommy, can we go to Disneyland?" the child asks. "Sure we can go, one of these days" comes the answer. The parents don't want to say "no", and they don't want to upset the kids. Maybe they even want, and intend to take the kids to Disneyland one of these days. Some parents maybe don't have any intention to, but they figure the kids will forget about the whole thing eventually.

This is how the weak side might use the idea of the future to persuade the judge. "Your Honor, I agree with the Strong side. We do need to lose weight and get into shape. I fully support the idea of diet and exercise, and I think we should definitely act on this plan. However, it's September and the holidays are just around the corner. Swimsuit season is way off. We will start our diet and exercise program one of these days, not now, but when the time is right." These are just some of the tools that the weak side uses to get his way. It is easy to see how the judge can be tricked by the weak side with all of these persuasive arguments he makes. Many times her mind is made up, and she won't even listen to the Strong side, if she lets him speak at all.

In the next chapter we will take a look at what the Strong side might say to refute the weak side's arguments before we make up our mind to which side we will give control of our future.

Key points

-In his quest to get control of us, the weak side uses some powerful tools, among them are:

-The self-image; How we are in real life should conform to the picture and description of ourselves that is stored in our minds.

-The comfort zone; we should avoid change in order to remain in familiar territory where we seem to be safe.

-Fear; Stay away from anything that causes this feeling because it might harm us.

-Pain and pleasure; get away from what seems like pain and embrace what feels like pleasure.

-The future; we should do it someday, but not today.

Chapter 4
WHY THE STRONG SIDE HAS
A
BETTER CASE

In the previous chapter we learned some of the methods the weak side uses to convince the judge to see things his way, and act according to his wishes. Some of them are quite powerful, and often achieve their desired effect. They have prevented us from achieving our goals in the past. The judge frequently decides without even considering the Strong side's case.

In this chapter we will finally give the Strong side his day in court. The Strong side will respond to each of the points raised by the weak side in an attempt to show how flimsy they truly are.

Self-image

The self-image, like all of our traits is a two-sided coin. It can either help us or hurt us. It's up to us to control it, just like shifting from reverse to forward in our car. We can't eliminate it, but we can use it to our benefit.

The trouble with the self-image is that it's not <u>real!</u> It's a figment of our imagination. It exists only in our minds. It's just a story that we make up about ourselves, and it is based on very bad, out-dated and obsolete evidence. It seems to be true because we rarely question it, so most of us accept it as fact when it's really just an illusion. Where does the self-image come from, and why does it seem real?

The self-image develops over the course of our lifetimes, but mostly during early childhood. As a child your mind was far more receptive to things. The child's mind accepts ideas without first questioning them. This is how young children learn so quickly. You learned to speak your native language, without actually being taught, in the first few years of life. If you have ever tried to learn a second language as an adult, you know how difficult it is.

The trouble with learning so quickly is that some false information is learned along with the true. Some of the things the self-image accepts as fact maybe were true of us at one time in our lives. Maybe something happened to us at five years of age that caused us to believe we were a certain way, or possessed a particular ability or inability. We formed a conclusion about ourselves, it was accepted as fact, and it was stored in our self-image and never thought of again. It might or might not have been true then, but we may still believe it now. Maybe we were clumsy and awkward at five years of age, so our grandfather, not meaning any harm, might have told us so. Not knowing any better at that age, we would have accepted it as a fact, and it became part of our self-image. Now at age 35 if you drop something you say "I'm so clumsy, I have always been a klutz."

The self-image contains hundreds and hundreds of examples like this that were valid at one time, but are no longer true. It also contains many more that were never true, but we still accept them as fact.

Because much of the self-image was developed during childhood, it still contains information that was put there by other children. You might have been on a playground somewhere at the age of six, and some nine-year-old might have called you "ugly" or "stupid" or "fat." When you are six, someone who is nine seems to be an authority. They were bigger and smarter and more experienced than you, so you believed what they said. Would you take seriously anything a nine-year-old said about you today? Of course not, it is only a child, but we still unconsciously believe what some kid said about us thirty years ago.

Almost invariably, the self-image does not match who we really are, and how others see us. Take for example the person who is afflicted with anorexia. We have all seen on television, at one time or other, the stories of people who suffer from this heart-breaking disease. It is plain to anyone looking at them that they are just skin and bones, but when they look at themselves in the mirror they see a fat person. This illustrates the power of the self-image, but also and more importantly, how wrong it can be and frequently is.

The good news about the self-image is that since it is just something that we made-up in the first place, a story that we created about ourselves as we were growing up, we can simply create a new and improved version now based on how we want to be. Once we create our new self image, we will begin to live up to it in the same way that we lived down to the old one that was holding us back for so long.

You created your current self-image, so that proves you have the power to create a new one. First, sit down and write out a description of the person that you want to be. Be as specific as possible in your description of this person. Second, read the description to yourself several times a day. As you do this, **convince yourself that is the <u>real you</u>**. Tell yourself that your new self-image is your **<u>normal</u>** condition.

Once you have successfully done this, your mind will want to "get back to normal." It will see your current physical condition as temporary and abnormal, and begin moving you in the direction that you want to be going.

This new self-image will be the one used as evidence when trying to get the judge to decide. When the question arises as to what to eat or not eat, refer to the new self-image and ask the judge what that person would do. Since that is the image of the real you, the judge would do right by matching your actions to those of the real you, instead of the inaccurate picture presented by the weak side.

Comfort zone

Think back to when you were just learning to drive a car. It probably felt very unnatural. The first time you were behind the wheel you didn't know how hard to push down on the gas or brake pedals to make the car go and stop smoothly. If you learned to drive in a car equipped with a manual transmission, it was twice as difficult. You did not have the "feel" for driving, and so you were not comfortable doing it.

If you have been driving for any amount of time, you can now do it without even thinking about it. Not only drive, but drink coffee, put on make-up, talk on your cell-phone and change the radio station all at the same time!

Do you remember your first day at your first or current job? You didn't know anybody, or how the company did things, or even where the bathroom was located. You didn't know who was nice or not so nice, so you kept quiet until you got the feel of the place. Now, after you have been there a while it seems like home. You have your personal space, maybe your own office or cubicle or work area with pictures of your family and friends.

These are just 2 of the many examples of things that were, at one time, outside of your comfort zone, but now are part of it. Some others include your first apartment, your first kiss, your first day at school, and your first time on an airplane.

If you had stayed within your comfort zone, you never would have done these things, or anything else new. Think of all the wonderful experiences that you would have missed-out on! And now, when you look back, you realize it was no big deal.

You once felt uncomfortable doing the things you do now because you didn't know what to expect. Once you did those things, your comfort zone expanded to include them. Your best friend was once a stranger whom you knew nothing about.

I can remember back when I was in grade-school and the first VCRs came on the market. I was so excited when my parents bought one a few years later. I quickly purchased a membership at a local video store that allowed me the privilege of renting their videos. I soon amassed a big collection of my own from movies and shows I had taped from the TV.

When DVDs came out, I had no interest in them. I was in my comfort zone with VHS. Why go out and get involved with this new format when I was perfectly content to keep things the way they were? If it isn't broken, don't fix it.

When they stopped selling movies on VHS, my comfort zone got very uncomfortable in a hurry. Now I had to get a DVD player so I could see the latest movies. When I go to the flea market and the thrift store now, and I see piles of VHS tapes that once cost anywhere from $19 to $99 when they were new, and they can't sell them for $1, they seem so primitive now that I can't believe I ever valued them so highly. The DVD has become normal, and the VHS has become abnormal.

Do you know anyone who stays in a bad relationship or keeps working at a job that they hate? The comfort zone is what keeps these people stuck where they are. They believe the old saying: "the devil you know is better than the devil you don't know." They think if they change jobs or mates that things might get worse. They are correct, things may get worse, but they also might get better. If they stay where they are at, things will never get any better, and will most likely get worse. Isn't it worth the risk to step out of the comfort zone?

The only sure-fire way to conquer the comfort zone is to just do the uncomfortable thing a few times. If you do, the comfort zone will expand and these things will soon become natural. If you don't, it will get smaller and you will miss-out on so many wonderful things that life has to offer. The only way to grow is to move beyond the boundaries of your comfort zone. Break out of that prison of your own making.

Fear

I could try to convince you that you must banish fear from your life. I could remind you that most fears never come true, and it's a wasted emotion. I could remind you of Franklin D. Roosevelt's immortal words "We have nothing to fear, but fear itself."

I could say all these things, but I have a better idea. For the purpose of this book, why not use fear to help us get what we want?

Here is what I mean…since we all have a certain amount of fear inside of us already, let's choose to fear the things we want to get away from. I am talking about things like heart disease, diabetes, high blood pressure, cholesterol, and all the other unpleasant things associated with being overweight. We can also include embarrassment, social stigma and general discomfort.

We should fear all of these things, but mostly we should fear the weak side. The weak side is the enemy. If he gets his way, we will lose.

When we use fear in this way, to get what we want, we turn a negative into a positive. Have you ever known anybody who had a medical scare that caused them to finally give up smoking, drinking, overeating or some other destructive habit? Their doctor used the power of fear to get them to change for the better. If it works, why not use it? The things I mentioned before are plenty of 100% legitimate things to be afraid of if you are overweight, so it does make perfect sense to fear them.

Pain

The same advice goes for pain as it does for fear; use it to your advantage. Has being overweight and out of shape ever caused you pain? Is it easy to live in an oversized body? Are you comfortable in your clothes, or out of them for that matter? Is it painful to climb stairs or exert yourself in any way? Do your feet or knees ever hurt due to excess weight?

Have you ever experienced emotional pain as a result of being too heavy? How many opportunities have you missed-out on? Has it ever contributed to the failure of a romantic relationship, or prevented one from starting in the first place? Have you ever felt self-conscious at the beach or in a social environment? I could go on, but I am sure you get the idea.

Now let me ask you this... which pain is worse, the pain of being overweight 24 hours a day, 7 days a week, 365 days a year, or the perceived pain of eating right and exercising that the weak side uses to prevent us from doing it? The answer is obvious.

I suggest you focus on the real pain, and move in the direction away from it. Move toward the pleasure of the body that you will have if you exercise and eat right. Diet and exercise lead to pleasure. Overeating and a sedentary lifestyle will only lead to more pain.

The future

The idea of doing it someday is such a common trap that people fall into that I have devoted an entire chapter to it called "The power of now." For right now though, let's just say the future is not here yet. In order to get what we want in the future, we must act now. The future is made out of the choices we make now.

As you can see, the Strong side has easily refuted all of the arguments, one by one, made by the weak side in the previous chapter. As if that weren't enough, let's look at some more compelling evidence in favor of the Strong side.

It's easier!

Have you ever noticed how problems seem to get worse and multiply when we put them off or try to avoid them? When we take the "easy way" or the quick fix it always winds-up costing us more time, money and trouble down the road. Then when we look back on it, we think "why didn't I just do it right to begin with?!"

Years ago, I worked for a man who owned several apartment and office buildings. Any time that a minor (or major) repair needed to be done, he would instruct me to do it in the cheapest way possible, instead of the right way. The proper action would cost only slightly more in the short term, and would have taken a bit more time now, but it would be fixed permanently. The shortcut would always end-up having to be fixed again and again and costing many times the money and time than if it had been fixed properly in the first place. This man was convinced he was doing things "the easy way," but it always turned-out to be "the hard way."

It's a funny thing, but many times in life the thing that seems like the easy way is really the hard way 99.99% of the time. The person who goes through life doing things the seemingly easy way is surely in for an up-hill battle. If we go through life doing things the way the weak side wants us to do them, our lives will be filled with trouble, pain and misery.

It is perfectly right and sensible to want to do things and live life the easy way. That is exactly what we are doing when we listen to the Strong side.

Living your life the Strong way is the easiest way!

Whom do you imagine has the easier (and longer) life, the overweight person, or the lean and healthy person? The one who exercises and eats right, or the one who eats junk food and sits on the sofa all day? The weak person, or the Strong one?

I am sure you know the answers to these questions. I am sure you know that the Strong way is truly the best way to live.

Key points

-The self-image is something we created in our imagination, so let's create one that helps us, instead of hurts us.

-The comfort zone will expand quickly if we do things outside of it. It will shrink if we do not.

-Use fear and pain as tools to get away from the things you don't want.

-The future is made from the decisions we make now.

-Strong is the easiest way to live.

.

Chapter 5
YOU BE THE JUDGE

So far, we have learned why we have failed in the past. We now know the difference between success and failure always boils down to a simple choice, or series of choices. We know what the weak side wants, and why he wants it. We know what the Strong side wants. And we know that all we have is now. It all comes down to this question; are we going to be weak or Strong now?

You've heard all the arguments. If you were the judge which side would you choose, weak or Strong? Which side seems like the easier way to live? Which side do you think will lead us to what we want? Which side will cause us less pain and more pleasure? Which side will make us feel better now, weak or Strong?

Before you answer, let me give you a hypothetical situation. What if your best friend or a special loved one came to you with a favor to ask. This person is overweight, and they want to get into shape. The person says "I will do whatever you say, I am putting myself in your hands, I hereby turn control of my life over to you." This person wants you to be their judge.

You agree to help them, and on the first day your friend calls you and asks "I am hungry, should I eat a bag of cookies or a salad?" They also ask "should I go to the gym or relax on the couch?" They tell you they prefer the cookies and couch, but you are the boss and they will do what you say and continue to love you either way.

What would you tell them to do? Would you have to spend a lot of time deciding? Remember, this person is counting on you. They love you and trust you so much that they have appointed you as their judge. Are you going to let them down, or will you have them do what you know is best for them?

Pretty easy choice, isn't it? But this is the exact same choice that comes up in our own minds, over and over again, when we are trying to lose weight. The only difference is that it's not your friend asking for help…it's **you!**

Earlier I said we all have a weak side, Strong side and a judge. Well, this may come as a surprise to you, and maybe some of you have already figured it out, but **you are the judge.** Yes you! The power to choose is in your hands. You and you alone, are in the driver's seat in your life. Just like how your friend in the above example gave control of his life over to you, you have absolute control of the decisions that govern your life. You are the judge, once you decide to do something, that's what you do. You have the power to choose, it is the greatest power that you possess.

Yes, you are in control of the decisions you make. You are where you are today as a direct result of the decisions that you have made in the past. Not your mother, father, kids, husband, wife or employer, just you. All of the skipped workouts and "just this once" junk food binges in the past are why you need to lose some weight now. The choices you make now will create the body you will have in the future.

It has been said that the more you do of what you have done, the more you will get of what you have gotten. In other words, the choices you have made in the past have gotten you to where you are now. If you want different results in the future, you must make different choices now.

You did not choose to be fat, but you did choose to do the things that resulted in your becoming and/or staying fat. Nobody else forced you to overeat or prevented you from exercising; you used the power of choice and decided to do so. It is the same power of choice that you must use now to do the things that will result in your becoming and staying lean, healthy and strong.

There are so many things in life that we have little or no control over; the weather, how tall we are, our ethnic background, the state of the economy, other people, how our favorite sports team performs, how lucky or un-lucky we are. All of these things are out of our hands. They are controlled by forces unknown and unaffected by us. But control over the decisions you make will always be yours.

You not only have total control of the actions you take or don't take, but you also have control of what you think. Nobody can make you think a certain way or believe something that you don't want to believe. If they could, everybody would think and act the exact same way. You choose your thoughts just as you choose your actions.

You can choose to think of things in a way that will either enhance or detract from the quality of your life. You can choose to believe that dieting is easy or difficult. You can believe exercising is fun and uplifting, or an unpleasant chore. You can choose your self-image. You can choose your own comfort zone. You can choose to believe that you can, and will be successful.

This amazing power of choice even extends to our emotions. You can choose to be happy or sad. You don't have to wait for a reason to feel any particular way; you have the power to choose to feel any way you wish at any time. Very few people make use of this ability or are even aware that they possess it.

I suggest you practice using the control of thought and feeling as soon and as often as possible so that you may develop the habit of thinking in a way that is empowering.

There is a lot of talk about "empowerment" nowadays. It seems like every time you turn on the television or open a magazine there is someone telling us about empowerment. What can be more empowering than using the power of choice to get what we want from life? It's more difficult to live a week life than it is to live a Strong one. It's easier to live Strongly and it feels good to live Strongly. It feels bad to live week. You have the power to choose.

I am completely in favor of empowerment. It feels good to be empowered, and it feels good to win. Conversely, it hurts to lose. Every time you chose to do what the Strong side wants, you win. Every time you give-in to the weak side you lose. You, and only you, have the power to turn the Strong side from a loser to a winner.

The weak side is the real enemy. You have the power to make sure he never again wins another case. Now that you know his tricks, and know that you are the judge, how can you let him win anymore? Remember that when weak loses, you win! The moment you start to feel tempted to cheat, you will realize that it is just the weak side trying to trick you again.

If you cheat on your diet, how does it make you feel afterward? Do you feel guilty or ashamed or weak? When you stay Strong don't you feel proud of yourself later? You deserve to feel that way.

You can either be your own worst enemy, or your own best friend. All you have to do is make a choice that only you can make. Choose the easy way! Choose the way that feels good! Choose Strong now!

In the past you thought you were choosing the easy way when you let the weak side win. The "easy way" was, in reality, the hard way (weak) in disguise. The truly easy way (Strong) appeared to be the hard way. The judge (you) was being tricked into making the wrong choice again and again. Refuse to be tricked ever again!

Feel good about choosing "Strong" because you know it is the right choice. Feel good about choosing "Strong" because it is the easiest way to live your life. Feel good every time the weak side loses another case. Feel proud every time you choose the Strong side over the weak.

This is the key that will open the lock to your treasure chest. Live this way and you will not only get the body you want, but just about anything else you desire from life.

Key points

-You are in total control of the decisions that you make in your life.

-Your past decisions have gotten you to where you are now.

-The decisions you make now will create your future conditions.

-In the past you thought "weak" was easy and "Strong" was hard.

-Now, in fact, you see that "Strong" is easy and "weak" is difficult.

Chapter 6
THE POWER OF NOW

Each of our lives is made up of a certain amount of this stuff we call time. Time is expressed in terms of the past, the present, and the future.

The past has already happened. It's over and done with. It exists only in our memory, and our memories tend not to be very accurate. They fade and alter what had really occurred based on emotion. My grandparents used to tell   me how wonderful everything   was back in the "good old days." To listen   to them you would think that the world was a paradise when they were young. But the fact is that life was much harder for them than they chose to remember. Time had distorted the truth in their memories.

Far too many people waste precious time and energy dwelling on what happened in the past. There is nothing you or I can do to change what has happened in the past. All we can do is learn from it and move on. The past does not equal the future. If you were a certain way last week, there is no law that says you have to be that same way next week.

The future hasn't happened yet, and is therefore uncertain by its nature. It exists only in our imagination. We don't know for sure what will happen tomorrow, next month, or next year so we must use our imagination when thinking of the future.

The future does not seem as real as the past because we have not seen it yet. That is why so many of us waste so much time dwelling in the past; we have already been there so it seems real. The problem is that living in the past will do nothing to shape our future.

When we set a goal for ourselves, it must take place in the future. The trouble is that we don't live in the future, we live now.

How many people do you know, or do you imagine there are who, in the beginning of the year, make so-called "New Year's resolutions"? There are millions of them. Now how many of them do you think break them before the year is over? How many before a month? How many don't last a week? I am sure you will agree that it is a very high percentage.

Why does this happen every year? Is there something wrong with each one of the good people who make New Year's resolutions? Of course not, but there is definitely something wrong with the process of making the New Year's resolution.

As I said earlier, we don't live in the future. We don't live one year at a time. It's impossible for the mind to grasp the idea of "I will do, or not do, something this year" because we don't live in one year increments.

We live now!

Our lives are really made up of infinitely small units of time called now. Now is the space of time between the past and the future.

Now is the only thing we have any real control over. If we want to get a certain outcome in the near future, for example, if we want to be somewhere in 10 minutes and it takes 10 minutes to get there, we better leave now. If we want to get there on time, we had better spend every one of the "nows" in-between here and there moving constantly in the right direction. This is clear and easy for our minds to understand, and it makes perfect sense.

But what if we stretch out our timeline to a year? "I want to lose 50 pounds this year." We have a whole year! That's a long time. "I can lose 50 pounds in a couple of months" you think. "If I lose 10 pounds a month, I could do it in five months standing on my head." It seems easy, so we think that we don't have to do anything now. "Surely, a piece of pie now is not going to stop me from losing 50 pounds this year."

What do you think will happen to this 50-pound goal by the end of the year? It will, most likely, remain unattained. The tendency is after the resolution is broken one time, it is usually forgotten about. Then we have to wait until next year to start over again.

The only difference between a year, and 10 minutes, is the amount of "nows" each one contains. Our entire lives are made-up of millions of "nows".

Think of a thirty-story brick building. All of those bricks had to be put into place one-at-a-time. They didn't just get there all at once. Each one of those bricks represents its own now. If the brick mason had gotten to the construction site on the first day of work and said to himself "I have plenty of time to build this wall, I think I will do something else now" the building would not be there today.

Brick+Brick+Brick=Building.
Just like;
Now+Now+Now=Your future and Your life.

The only way to get what you want in the future is to do something now. Right now! Not tomorrow, or next Monday, or next month, or even in five minutes, Right Now. Now is all you really have. There is no need to wait until New Year's Eve to make a resolution, make a **now** resolution!

The closer your resolution is to now, the more powerful it is. A now resolution is stronger than a 3 o'clock resolution. A 3 o'clock resolution is stronger than a 4 o'clock resolution. A 4 o'clock resolution has more power than a tomorrow resolution, and so on.

As the judge, you must not let the weak side have control of now. Whichever side (weak or Strong) gets control of now wins. The weak side will attempt to treat you like a child and say "we will do it someday" in order to placate you and hope you will forget about it in time. You must not let this happen!

A good way to keep the weak side from getting control over now is to use his own tactics against him. Say "I will be weak someday, but I will be Strong now." And we all know that someday never comes.

Instant gratification

People tend to want results now. If someone offered you $100 now or $200 next month, I bet most people would choose the $100 now. A bird in the hand is worth two in the bush. The bird in the hand represents now.

Credit cards are so popular because they make use of the power of now. Buy now, pay later. If we are walking through the mall, and we see something in the window that we might not really need, but want now, we are more willing to buy it if we can charge it than if we had to pay cash. Money seems more valuable now than in the future when the bill comes due. We know that we will have to pay the bill someday, but it is in the future so it doesn't feel so bad. It doesn't have the power of now. That's why credit cards are a multi-billion dollar industry. It is also why merchants are willing to pay a percentage of each sale to the credit card companies. They realize that the power of now will increase sales more than enough to compensate for it.

We all want to feel good now. If we could exercise one time and get the body we want, or skip dessert one time and instantly lose 10 pounds, everyone would do it. But we all know it doesn't work that way. It takes time for our bodies to change. The body we want is in the future. Our desire to feel good and eat dessert is now. Just like with the credit card, it seems like the best way to feel good now is to eat the desert now, and pay for it later.

It is this trait which accounts for the popularity of liposuction and stomach stapling surgeries that are common today. People could simply eat less and exercise more to lose weight, but they opt for risky, expensive surgical procedures in order to get instant gratification.

There are billions of dollars spent each year on dubious, often dangerous pills and potions that promise instant, effortless weight-loss. The claims are too good to be true, but the desire for instant results is too strong, and it overrides common sense.

The weak side of our mind uses the "feel-good now, pay later" tactic to get its way all the time. All we have to do is associate feeling good now with doing what the Strong side wants. We know the Strong side is what's best for us, so doing what it wants now equals pleasure. We know that doing what the weak side wants equals pain in the future. Whenever we do what it wants it should make us feel pain.

Being weak now = pain
Being Strong now = pleasure

Whichever side, weak or Strong, is in control of now wins, that side has all the power. If this is our mindset, we will get what we want 100% of the time. The same power that has kept us from our goals in the past will now propel us towards them. We will want to eat right now, just as strongly as we wanted to eat junk food in the past. It will make us feel good now to go to the gym, just as it did in the past to loaf around the house and be a couch potato.

Remember our car's engine always turns in the same direction, whether we are going in reverse or forward. If we want to change the direction we are traveling in, we don't try to change the direction of the engine, we simply shift gears.

When we let weak have control of now, we are going in reverse. By giving control of now to the Strong side we are shifting gears into drive. The moment you do this you start to move in the direction of your goals.

The prisons are full of people who choose to give control to their weak sides in order to feel good now. Think about it for a moment. If the criminal wants some money he thinks "what's the best way for me to get it now?" He concludes that stealing it is a good idea, disregarding the consequences. Or take for example the drug user. He thinks "what's the best way for me to feel good now?" Take some drugs is his answer. Or the rapist who thinks "what's the best way for me to feel sexual gratification now?" Even the murderer who, for whatever reason, wants to see the other guy dead, kills him to feel good now. For these people jail seemed less important, less real, (because it may or may not be in the future) than what they wanted now (at the time they committed their crimes).

Everyone wants to feel good now, and I want you to as well. It is in our nature to want this, and that is why denying one's self seldom works. It's like trying to get our engine to run backwards to get the car to go in reverse. Eventually the perceived pain of self-denial becomes so great that we choose to do what the weak side wants in order to feel good now. All we have to do is choose to feel good about being Strong now, and feel badly about being weak now. That's all there is to it. And it sure does feel good to be Strong now, just as it feels bad to be weak. Because we now know that Strong is the easiest and the correct way to live.

Another industry that makes use of the power of now is the "rent-to-own" industry. They cater to people who have poor credit and low incomes. If you want a new TV that costs $500, for example, but don't have $500, they will rent you one to use now. After you have paid the rent for a certain period of time, it becomes yours. The problem is that by the time you finish paying, you've probably paid about $1500 to $2000 for the $500 TV. That's the power of now.

Still another very lucrative industry that makes use of the power of now is the "cash advance" or "payday loan" business. These people will loan you money for a very short-term (until payday) and a very high rate of interest.

People are willing to pay extra now to get a portion of their paycheck, rather than wait until payday to get the full amount.

The states that have lotteries use the same principal to get money from their people. They used to have a drawing once or twice a week until they figured out they could make more money by offering instant scratch-off tickets. Some states have a keno game that plays every 10 minutes. People sit there all day and watch the numbers come up on a TV screen in hopes of instant money.

As you can see, these industries that depend on the power of now tend to cater to people who are in the weakest positions financially and emotionally. Also, dealing with them will tend to keep these people in that same condition for an even longer period of time than if they avoided them. How will they ever become financially sound if they keep paying these exorbitant interest rates, or spending money they can't afford on lottery tickets that offer almost no chance of winning?

I am not condemning these industries. What they do is legal and there is a demand for it. Also, they deal with high-risk customers. Some of them might rent the TV, pay the first month, and then disappear and never make another payment. Maybe they will sell the TV or move to a different address. This is the justification for the high interest rates. Furthermore, people don't have to do business with them if they don't choose to. I only bring them up to illustrate; 1) the power of now, 2) human tendency to want to feel good now regardless of future circumstances, and 3) how this very tendency is a vicious cycle that will only keep us in the weak condition indefinitely.

This is the exact situation we face when dieting; 1) we want to feel good now. 2) so we decide to eat a half of a pie a-la-mode now, thinking that we will make up for it in the future by eating less tomorrow and working-out twice as hard next week, until 3) eventually we get in over our heads, and give-up on our diet altogether.

Key points

-The past is gone forever. The future is uncertain. Now is all we have.

-The only way to secure your future is to do something now.

-People place a higher value on feeling temporarily good now, than feeling permanently good in the future.

-Decide to feel good now every time you   chose   to be   Strong.   Being Strong is its own reward.

Chapter 7
PUTTING IT ALL TOGETHER

As we go about our busy, 21st century lives it becomes very easy to forget the things we learn. We are bombarded by so much information in these modern times via books, newspapers, magazines, television, the internet etc. that the mind hasn't got the time to process it all.

In order to cope with all the demands we put on it, the mind develops "shortcuts" or automatic responses to the variety of situations that come up every day. This is where habits and knee-jerk reactions come from. If someone sneezes, you automatically say "bless you," even if you are not religious. If someone sticks out his hand to shake yours, you extend yours in return. If you are approached by a sales person you say "just looking" or "I'm not interested." If a scary-looking character is walking towards you on a dark, deserted street you cross to the other side.

We all do things like this. Not always the same things, but things we all do without having to consciously think about them. There are simply not enough hours in the day to have to consciously evaluate our every single move that we make.

In order for you to remember what you have read in this book, and make it a part of your life, I would like to suggest the following; get yourself a 3x5 index card and write on it "WEAK OR STRONG NOW?" Carry the card with you every day. If, at any time, you feel yourself wanting to cheat on your diet, or skip an exercise session, look at the card and ask yourself that simple but powerful question. I call it "the magic question."

Do not just write "be strong" or "don't be weak" as this lacks the full impact of "weak or Strong now?" This phrase is powerful because it concisely shows what we want to get away from (weak) and what we want to move towards (Strong). It also incorporates time (now) into the equation, so it prevents us from postponing the decision. If you catch yourself procrastinating, recognize it as the weak side trying to trick you again, and refuse to be tricked.

This simple four-word question is the essence of the philosophy of this book.

WEAK

This word represents failure, loss, pain and shame. This is the opposite of what we want. We know we must avoid it at all cost. Weak is the enemy. It is trying to prevent us from getting what we want, just as it has done to us so many times before.

OR

This word reminds us that the choice is ours. We are in control. We are in the driver's seat in our own life, and there is nobody in the entire world who can take this power from us.

STRONG

This is the easy way to live. This is what we want because it is right and good. Every time we choose "Strong", we win instantly. When we win we feel pride and empowerment. These feelings are far more satisfying than anything the weak side has to offer.

NOW

Not later, but <u>right this second</u>. This is the time for a decision. If you don't make a decision to be Strong now, you are in fact deciding to be weak by default.

When you ask yourself this question in this way, it is very difficult to actually choose "weak." There are only 2 choices, "weak" or "Strong". It's like choosing between good or bad, right or wrong, pain or joy. If you do not choose "Strong" now, you automatically choose "weak" by default. There is no in-between; it is always either "weak" or "Strong".

I think it's safe to say most people will choose "Strong" every time. In the extremely unlikely event that you should ever choose "weak", it's not the end of the world. It is not an excuse to give-up on the whole idea. Just start again with the very next decision that you face.

If you do happen to choose "weak", it will make you that much more likely to choose "Strong" the next time. It does not feel good to choose to be weak. It does feel good and empowering to choose to be Strong. This will be the source of your instant gratification from now on, instead of fattening foods and inactivity.

To reinforce this further, on the other side of the card I would like for you to write a pledge to yourself that you will always choose "Strong" over "weak". This pledge can be anything you choose to write that will motivate you. It doesn't have to be long, a few sentences will do. After you write it, sign it and date it to make it official.

Another good way to increase your chances of success is to involve someone else to act as a helper for you, and you for them. It should be someone whom you trust, and see often. A spouse or close relative is ideal because they want you to succeed as much as you do.

I suggest you have them read a copy of this book first so they are familiar with its concepts. (Additional copies are available on our web site, www.simplesecretbook.com) After they have read it, make an agreement with them that you will help them to choose "Strong", and they will help you to do the same. It will be much harder to ever choose "weak" with another person involved as you don't want to look inconsistent with your pledge in their eyes. It's also easier to choose "Strong" with their support and help in keeping you reminded of your goals.

It is of vital importance to keep reminding yourself throughout the day of this question; "weak or Strong now?" It is for this reason that we have made available on our web site some tools that will help to keep you reminded. We have refrigerator magnets, jewelry, water bottles, t-shirts etc. with the magic question printed on them so as to keep it at the forefront of your thinking. After a short period of time of having to ask yourself the magic question, your mind will develop a shortcut. You will begin to choose "Strong" automatically! You will no longer have to think about it. If someone asks you if you want cake, "no" will be your automatic reply. When it comes time to exercise, you will do it gladly because you actually want to. You won't have to force yourself. Nobody has to force themselves to do the things that they want to do.

I challenge you to begin this way of life right now, in fact I dare you to! I have 100% confidence in your ability to make the right choices and to succeed. I am sure this method will work for you if you will try it, and I look forward to hearing your success story. Don't let me down.

One more thing to keep in mind as you go along; this is the only life you have got to live. Do you really want to spend it living inside a body that is un-healthy, un-attractive and un-comfortable? The weak side does. Each time you decide in his favor, you agree to stay trapped in there a little while longer.

Key points

-It is vital to keep yourself reminded of what you have read here, and put it into practice.

-Write the magic question "weak or Strong now?" on a card and carry it with you. Read it several times a day, and if you ever feel that you may be slipping. Also, attach one to your refrigerator door and bathroom mirror.

-Enlist the help of a close friend or relative. Make a promise to each other to aid in choosing "Strong" over "weak".

-You can do it, I am counting on you!

Chapter 8
BEYOND WEIGHT-LOSS

As I stated in the introduction, this book was written primarily to aid the individual who is trying to lose weight and get into shape. It was done-so because of the great many people who fall into this category but it is, by no means, limited to them. This very same method can be employed to achieve practically anything you want within your capability.

The weak side/Strong side principal comes into play in many different areas of your life that you might not have realized, but can be just as useful when applied to them as it is when used for weight-loss.

Let's imagine, for instance, that you desire more money to better care for yourself and your family now and in the future. This is certainly a noble and worthwhile goal. No matter how much we have, we always seem to need more.

Now you and I know that to make and accumulate a lot of money we need to do certain things, and not do other things. These might include, but are not necessarily limited to;

-Getting a better education, perhaps earning an advanced degree.

-Working harder and more enthusiastically at our current job in order to advance in our career.

-Maybe getting a second job to supplement our income.

-Saving every extra dollar.

-Investing prudently every dollar that we do save.

All of the aforementioned would be classified in the "Strong" side. They might appear to be difficult now, but over the long term they are the easiest way to live.

We also know that to get rich we must avoid things like;

-Squandering money on frivolous things that we don't need like jewelry, designer anything (cloths, shoes, luggage, sunglasses etc.) electronic devices etc.

-Eating out in restaurants every day.

-Doing as little as possible at work, just enough to not get fired.

-Spending (wasting) our free time hanging-out in a bar.

-Looking for something for nothing.

All of these things would fall under the weak side. They might seem like fun now, but when you look back on your life 20 years from now with nothing to show for it, and no money saved-up, you will realize that you took the hard way. If you had followed the truly easy way, you could have amassed a small fortune in 20 years time, and could well afford to live comfortably for the rest of your life.

The weak side will use the same tricks he used in keeping you fat as he does in keeping you poor. Deal with them the same way. Whenever you have to decide on whether or not to buy some overpriced trinket or put the money into investments ask yourself "weak or Strong now?" If an opportunity comes up at work to go the extra mile and maybe impress your boss into giving you a raise and a promotion, but it might cut into your leisure time, ask yourself the magic question "weak or Strong now?"

If you are a parent and wish to be a better one, use the magic question. It takes work and time and patients to be a good parent, but what more important job is there? As a parent you make choices and decisions every day. When they come up, ask yourself the magic question. When your children get on your nerves and you feel frustrated and about to snap, stop for a moment and ask yourself the magic question.

If you really wish to be an outstanding parent, teach your children to live by the principals described in this book. If they start now, it will develop into a habit that will serve them well for the rest of their lives. Teach them to make the right choices and praise them when they do. This will not only make them better people, but it will make you a better person too.

Every time you help another person, be it a child or an adult, to choose "Strong" over "weak", you help yourself because you reinforce the idea by teaching it to others. When you hear the words come from your own voice and see the positive results that they have on others, the ideas will solidify in you and become a natural way of life for you, not to mention the personal satisfaction you will receive from helping others. It truly is better to give than to receive.

If you are not a parent, surely you know someone who could benefit from these principals. It's easy to see weakness in others that they might not even realize they have. There are many who feel helpless in life and think there is nothing they can do to change, so they don't even try. You know better than that. You can teach and inspire this person, and you will both benefit as a result.

If you are a religious or spiritual person, you can apply these concepts to that area of your life as well. It does not matter what your particular faith happens to be. There will always be times when you are faced with choices that go against the teachings of your church. When faced with situations like this, recognize that it is the weak side trying to fool your judge into making the wrong choice. As soon as you do, it will become easy for you to take the right path. If there is something in your life that you have been putting-off for a while, but needs doing, ask yourself the magic question. Maybe you need to go to the dentist or get a physical check-up. Do you need to apologize to someone to whom you have done wrong? How about visiting an old friend or loved one with whom you may have lost touch? Is there something you have always wanted to learn, or a project you have been meaning to start?

As you can see, there are countless situations in life, beyond weight-loss, that this same system can be applied to. Simply identify what it is that you want to do. Make a list of "weak side" excuses that have been keeping you from doing it so you will recognize them should they appear. Make a list of "Strong side" reasons why you should do this thing. And finally ask yourself that magic question; "weak or Strong now?"

Chapter 9
QUESTIONS AND ANSWERS

Q; What is the best type of exercise program to follow?

A; The best type of exercise program to follow is the one that you stick with! That being said, here are some guidelines that I recommend;

1) It must be challenging.

In order for the body to change, it needs something to respond to, or it will have no reason to change. Physical exercise works on the principal stimulus and response. If I were to lift weights today, for example, it would place a certain amount of stress on my muscles. My body would say to itself "if he does this again I better be ready", so it will release chemicals (hormones) into the blood that will cause my muscles to grow stronger. The actual process of exercise is a breaking-down of tissue, and the rest period in between exercise is a repair phase where the body builds itself back up to compensate. The same is true for running, swimming, stretching etc. the body is constantly adapting to stimulation, but it needs a real challenge to adapt to.

I am not saying that you have to "kill yourself" and risk injury. Over-doing it will only make matters worse, but you do have to work up a sweat and you should be breathing heavy. If it feels easy and comfortable you aren't exercising. If you go for a 20 minute walk, it's not going to stimulate any changes in your body unless you are hundreds of pounds overweight or you are walking up the side of a steep mountain. Obviously the amount of stimulation you need depends on how fit you are. If it has been a while since you have worked-out, or if you have never exercised before, **start slow!** Be honest with yourself and use common sense. Challenge yourself but don't strain or push too hard.

* Be sure to check with your doctor before beginning an exercise program*

2) Do something every day.

It is better to exercise 30 for minutes every day than for 3 hours once a week. You should do something different each day as well, to give the body time to recover from the previous day (ex. run Monday, swim Tuesday, weights Wednesday etc.) The body adapts quickly so it needs variety or it will stop and refuse to change if you do the same kind and amount of exercise every day.

3) Build some muscle

The more muscle you have, the more fat your body will burn. Also muscle gives your body it's shape, makes you strong, wards off illness, and generally contributes to overall good health.

A lot of ladies fear that muscle will make them lose their femininity and they will look like men. This is a myth. Building muscle will not make you look like a man. Your body chemistry will not allow this to happen, I promise. Building muscle will only enhance your natural femininity.

4) Short is better than long

To burn fat and build muscle, it is better to keep work-outs short but intense. For example, it would be better to sprint for 1 minute, rest for 1 minute, etc. for 15 minutes than it would to slowly jog for 30 minutes. This type of exercise is more effective at stimulating the body into making the kind of changes we want. The exercise program that I personally use and have found to be best is found on our web site; WWW.SIMPLESECRETBOOK.COM.

Q; Is it better to join a gym or work-out at home?

A; It depends on your personality and lifestyle, but I prefer home. I have belonged to many gyms over the years, and they have some good points, but I feel that I can get just as good of a work-out at home with minimal equipment.

When you exercise at home, you can do it whenever you want, it's more convenient than having to drive across town during the hours of operation of the gym. Also, there is no waiting to use equipment (that may or may not be clean), you don't have to think about who is looking at you or what you are wearing etc., and you can use your own bathroom! Furthermore, you will have one less excuse not to work-out if you do so at home ("I don't feel like going to the gym") Check the web site for some fine exercise equipment.

Q; You say that every diet works if you follow it, but are some better than others?

A; I made that statement to illustrate the point that when people fail at dieting, it's usually because they quit, not because the diet doesn't work. Some diets do indeed work better than others. On the web site you will find the one that I personally recommend. Choose a diet that will work best for you, with your lifestyle and food preferences. If you don't cook, choose one that features prepared food. If you can't live without meat, go low-carb. But the main thing is to stick with it!

Q; I see lots of advertisements for diet pills, food supplements and herbal remedies that make claims of easy weight-loss. What do you think of them?

A; I am in favor of using anything that works. If there is some tool available to help you reach your goal, I am all for it. The problem is that a lot of what you see advertised simply does not work. Only deal with reputable companies. If the claims seem too good to be true, they probably are. On the other hand, science is always making new discoveries. Keep an open mind. Maybe you know someone who has had success with one of these products. If so, give it a try and maybe it will work for you too. If I should hear of anything promising, I will post it on the website.

Q; I have been dieting successfully for almost a month now, but I get distracted easily because I am so busy and I find myself slipping into my old habits. How can I stop this?

A; Enlist the help of a friend. Talk often to this person about your success, but don't say that you are slipping. Only say that you are succeeding and it will become a part of you. Focus on the outcome that you want. Also, keep the magic question in your mind. Place it on sticky notes in locations that you will be sure to see it, like your computer monitor, bathroom mirror, refrigerator etc. Do this, and you will be surprised at how soon you will form the habit of success.

A Final Word of Thanks

I would like to take a moment now to sincerely thank you for reading this book. Even though we do not know each other personally, I truly wish my humble words will help and inspire you to make a positive change in your life. I know you will succeed if you give it a try, and I wish you all the luck in the world on your journey through life.

Sincerely,
B.T. Christopher

WWW.SIMPLESECRETBOOK.COM

www.ingramcontent.com/pod-product-compliance
Lightning Source LLC
Chambersburg PA
CBHW060906280326
41934CB00007B/1202